AMERICA

Scenic Wonders and Remarkable Sites
that Celebrate the Spirit of a Nation

An Interactive Book for Memory-Impaired Adults

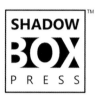

Shadowbox Press books are designed to facilitate a rewarding reading experience by providing entertainment, education, and comfort to individuals diagnosed with Alzheimer's disease, Parkinson's disease, stroke, brain injury, or other memory-impairment condition.

For more information, go to www.shadowboxpress.com

Shadowbox Press, established in 2009, is an independent publisher committed to providing high-quality, interactive books to the memory-impaired adult audience.

Published by Shadowbox Press, LLC
P.O. Box 268
Richfield, OH 44286
www.shadowboxpress.com

Chief Creative Director: Matthew Schneider
Product Development Director: Deborah Drapac, BSN, RN

This book is intended to be informational and should not be considered a substitute for advice from a health care professional. The authors and the publisher expressly disclaim responsibility for any adverse effects arising from the use or application of the information contained in this book.

Publisher's Cataloging-in-Publication data

Schneider, Matthew John.
    America : Scenic wonders and remarkable sites that celebrate the spirit of a nation, an interactive book for memory-impaired adults / Matthew Schneider ; Deborah Drapac, BSN, RN.
    p. cm.
    ISBN-13: 978-0-9831577-0-0; ISBN-10: 0-9831577-0-7
1. Alzheimer's disease—Patients—Rehabilitation. 2. Dementia—Patients—Rehabilitation.
3. Caregivers. 4. Self-care, Health. I. Drapac, Deborah Ann. I. Title.

RC523.S37 2011
362.196'831—dc22   2010917057

Manufactured in China

AMERICA

Scenic Wonders and Remarkable Sites that Celebrate the Spirit of a Nation

An Interactive Book for Memory-Impaired Adults

Matthew Schneider
Deborah Drapac, BSN, RN

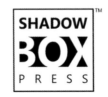

Shadowbox Press, LLC
Richfield, Ohio

INTRODUCTION

Shadowbox Press began with one simple mission: to develop interactive products for memory-impaired adults to revisit and share memories through the reading experience.

Storytelling is a valuable form of communication that connects one another and allows us to relate to each other on a personal level. It sparks the imagination, promotes self-reflection, and provides a way to find meaning in our experiences.

We have published a collection of books that offer a variety of subject matter designed to engage the user with meaningful content and provide a connection to both the past and present. Every effort has been made in the development of these books to maximize the experience for the user. They may be read independently or shared with an individual by a caregiver, loved one, staff member, or volunteer.

Our books offer a rewarding reading experience that stimulates the mind and offers engagement opportunities for the user. You will find inspiring words, inviting photographs, innovative conversation prompts, and unique activities to facilitate an interactive, multi-sensory experience. These books can generate meaningful communication and provide the feeling of well-being associated with sharing experiences and stories together. Through engagement, you may discover common backgrounds and interests, realize mutual bonds, and/or participate in a quality conversation.

We believe the reading experience should be shared at all stages of life, and sincerely hope that our passion for books touches your heart. We trust that you will find meaning, delight, and comfort in sharing a title from our collection of Shadowbox Press books. May you explore and discover memories, share experiences, and reflect on the value and purpose of life.

At Shadowbox Press, we welcome feedback from our readers and listeners. Please contact us at www.shadowboxpress.com to share your reading experiences, stories, and suggestions for future books.

ABOUT THIS BOOK

This book has been created to provide an interactive reading experience for a memory-impaired adult. It is designed to encourage socialization, evoke memories, prompt conversation, and supply mental and physical stimulation, thereby improving the overall quality of life for the individual user.

There are a variety of benefits from using this book. By encouraging engagement through personal reminiscing, a feeling of empowerment, an elevated mood, a positive self-image, and/or a reduced level of depression may result. In addition, a caregiver's presence, support, and attention can communicate acceptance, reassurance, and affection to a memory-impaired adult.

This book is comprised of three sections:

1. The STORY is the foundation of the book and is designed to entertain, inform, inspire, and/or educate. It features inviting photographs paired with engaging, large-print text written in clear, concise, and easy-to-read sentences. The content is intended to cultivate an interest in reading, evoke memories, and encourage opportunities to reminisce.

2. CONVERSATION STARTERS are questions that directly correlate to an individual set of pages from the STORY. Each series of inquiry-based questions are designed to prompt a dialog from experiences, events, and/or relationships. Engaging in conversation provides a memory-impaired adult the opportunity to share special memories and unique experiences from their life.

3. ACTIVITIES are exercises based on sensory stimulation, creative expression, and physical movement. These simple but purposeful activities correspond to the overall theme of the book, and are designed to provide additional mental and physical enrichment. Participation in a variety of activities is essential to overall good health and emotional well-being.

This book does not have to be read in its entirety to provide a benefit. Each set of pages is intended to encourage thinking, stimulate emotions, and evoke unique memories. An individual page may trigger a response and lead to a meaningful conversation. Through the reading and reminiscing process, the user can share his or her unique life story, express personal values, and, perhaps, reveal a legacy to pass on to future generations.

INTERACTION GUIDELINES

Communication is what connects us to each other. Because memory impairment slowly diminishes communication skills, it creates distinct challenges in how an individual communicates their thoughts and emotions, as well as comprehend what is being communicated to them. The key to managing the behaviors associated with memory impairment lies in the methods of engagement by caregivers and others. It is important to adapt our thinking and behaviors to create a more comfortable environment for a memory-impaired adult.

Guidelines for a successful reading experience:

- Locate a quiet, comfortable setting, free of distractions, for the reading experience.
- Before beginning, take a moment and allow yourself to relax. Imagine a connection between the voice and the story and reflect upon the importance of the time spent together.
- Always approach the individual from the front and make eye contact.
- Position your head at the same level as the individual's head. Bend your knees or sit down to reach a correct level.
- Smile whenever it's appropriate. A connection can grow from a smile.
- Present the book to the individual and invite them to share in the reading experience.
- Read aloud slowly, in an adult tone with a clear, calm, inviting, and enthusiastic voice, pausing after each sentence.
- Speak in short, direct sentences, focusing on a single idea at a time.
- Focus on central words and ideas, emphasizing the ones that may evoke memories.
- Point out key aspects of the photographs and invite the individual to share their thoughts.
- Include your own comments and encourage the individual to share their memories by prompting them with the CONVERSATION STARTERS.
- Ask only one question at a time, allowing the individual to answer it before continuing.
- Be aware of nonverbal cues. It is often possible to recognize a connection by observing facial expressions and/or body language.
- After a response, either verbal or nonverbal, acknowledge the contribution with positive reinforcement and encourage further discussion.
- Remember to be patient, as it may take longer for a memory-impaired adult to fully process and respond to a particular word, phrase, idea, or image.
- At times, engagement may become challenging. However, always treat the individual with dignity and respect.

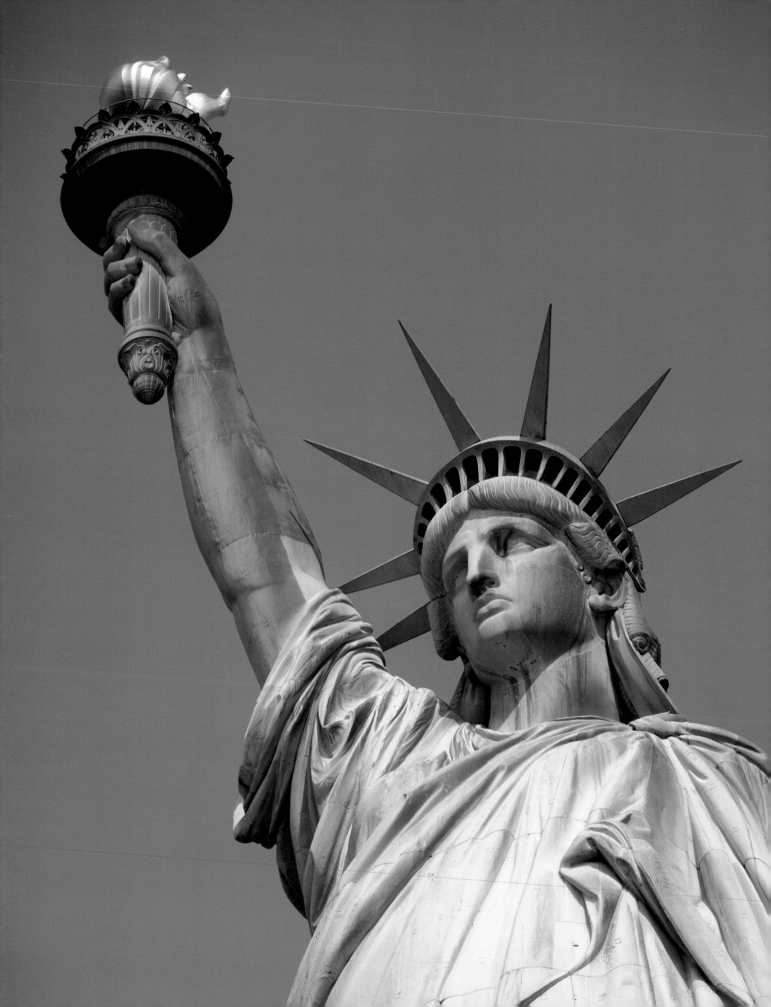

Statue of Liberty

New York, New York

The Statue of Liberty is located in New York Harbor. It was a gift of international friendship from the people of France. Dedicated on October 28th, 1886, it remains a universal symbol of democracy.

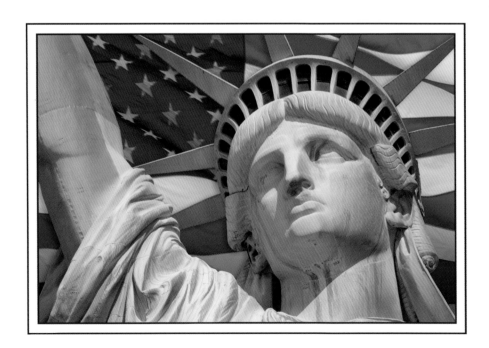

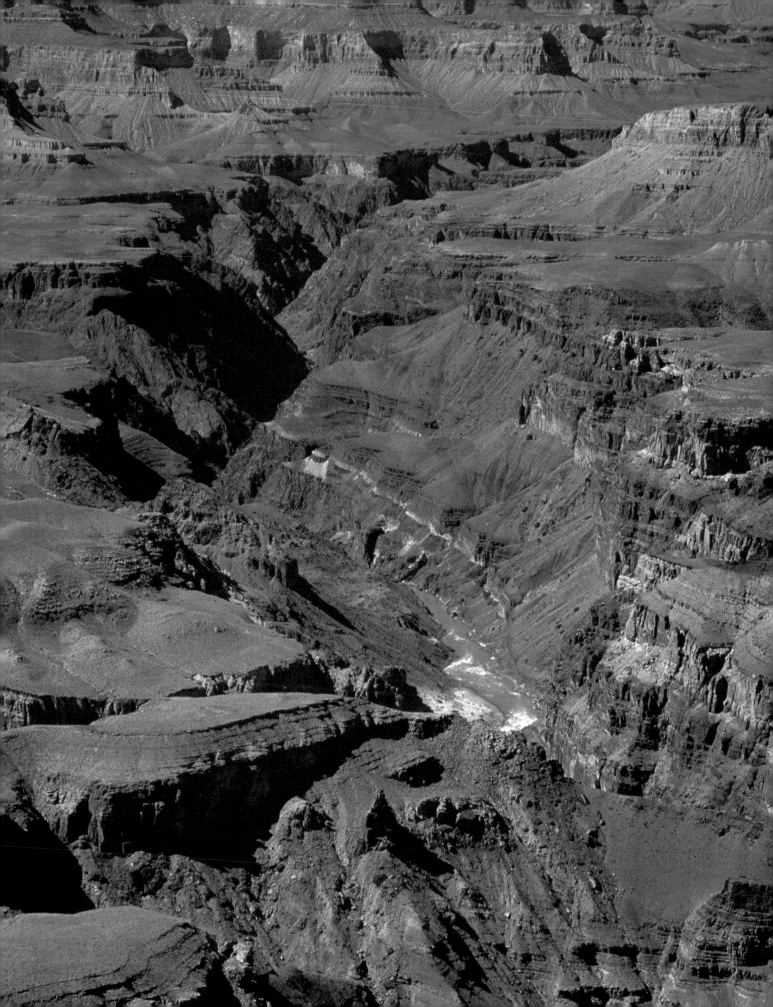

Grand Canyon

Arizona

The Grand Canyon is an enormous gorge created by the Colorado River. It covers over one million acres and is one of the natural wonders of the world. Best known for its amazing size and beautifully colored landscape, the Grand Canyon is one of the world's most popular sightseeing destinations.

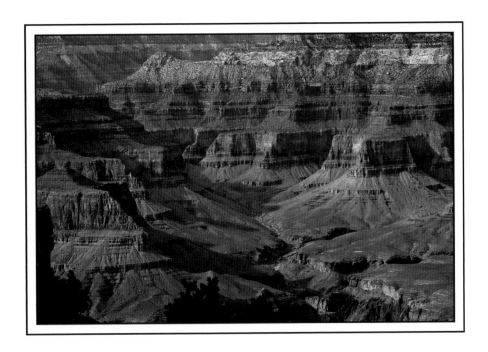

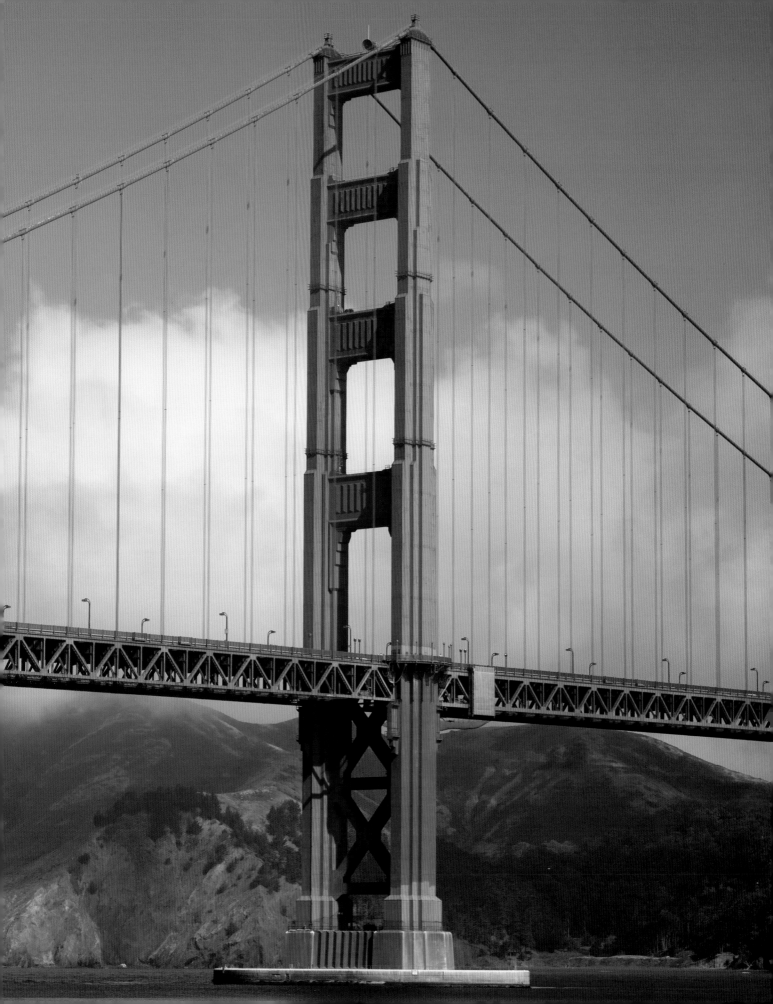

Golden Gate Bridge

San Francisco, California

The Golden Gate Bridge spans the entrance
to the San Francisco Bay. This engineering
marvel, with its tremendous towers
and sweeping cables, is considered one
of the world's most beautiful bridges.

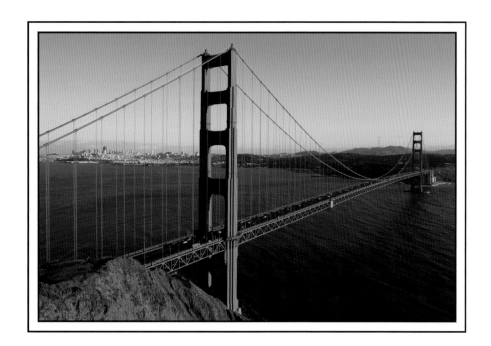

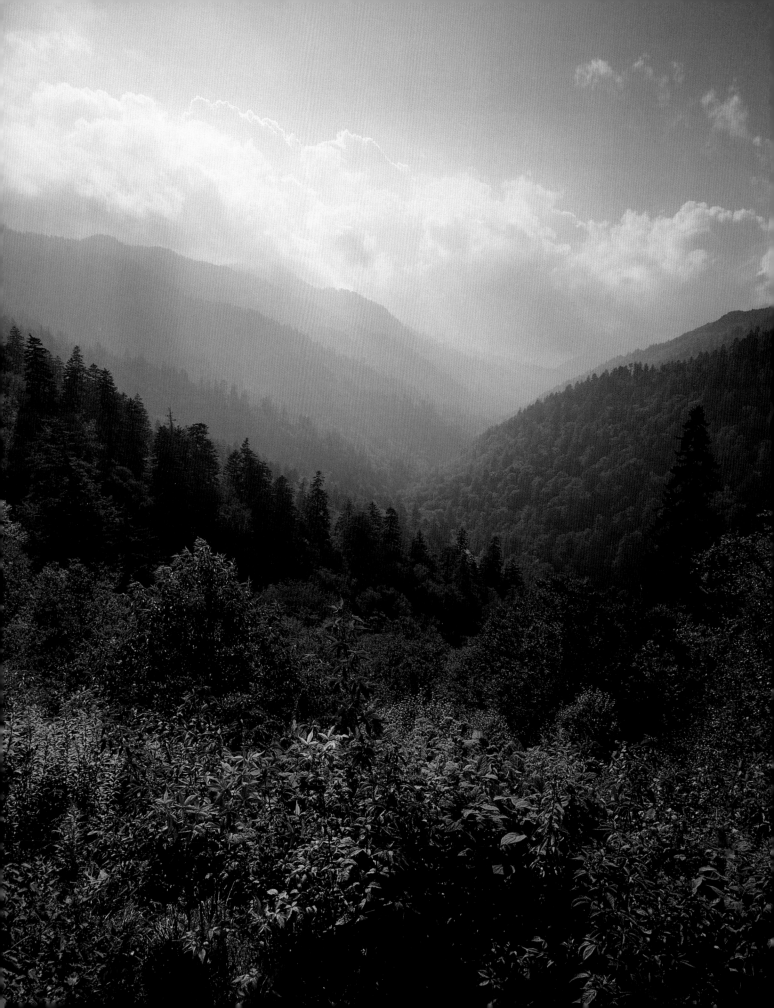

Great Smoky Mountains

Tennessee

The Great Smoky Mountains are named
for the smoke-like haze that envelops them.
One of its most popular lookout spots
is Clingman's Dome. With an elevation
of 6,643 feet above sea level, it's the highest
point in Tennessee.

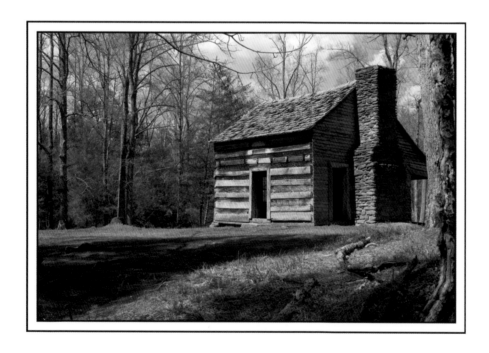

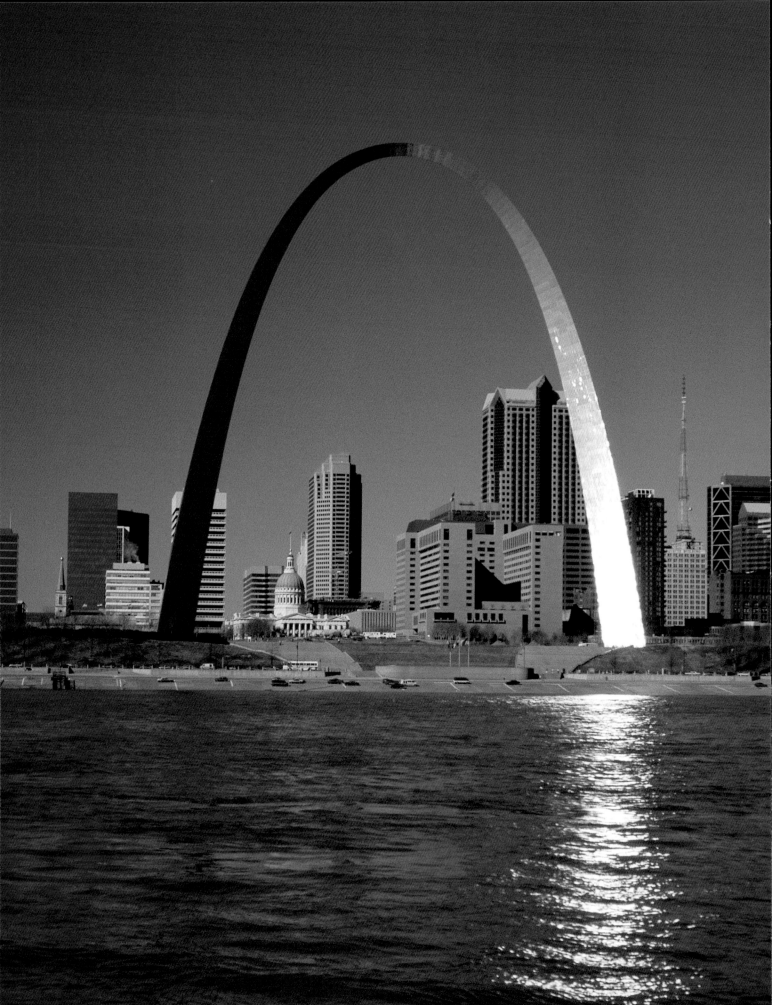

Gateway Arch

St. Louis, Missouri

The Gateway Arch is the tallest monument in the United States. The 630-foot high, stainless steel arch was built as a memorial to the expansion of the United States across the North American continent.

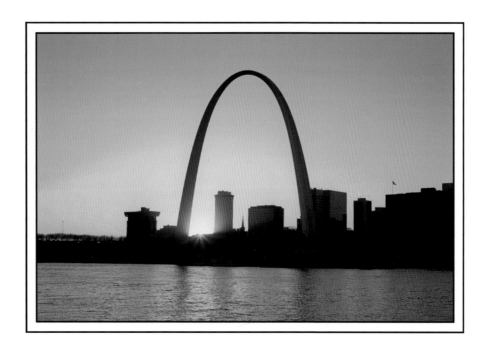

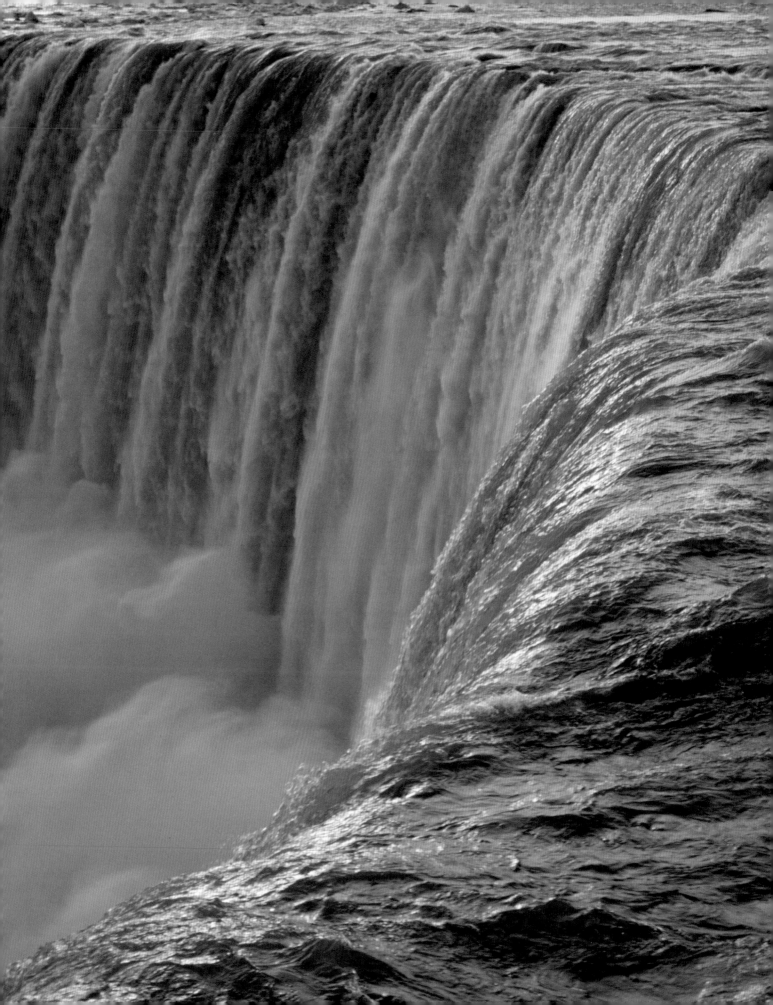

Niagara Falls

United States, Canada

Niagara Falls is comprised of two major sections.
The Horseshoe Falls are located on the Canadian
side of the border, while the American Falls,
and much smaller Bridal Veil Falls, are on
the United States side. Niagara Falls is a valuable
source of hydroelectric power, and is considered
one of the most awesome natural wonders
in North America.

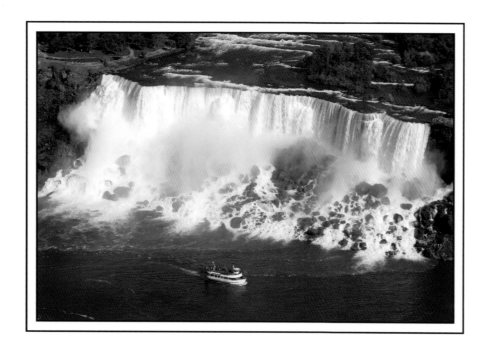

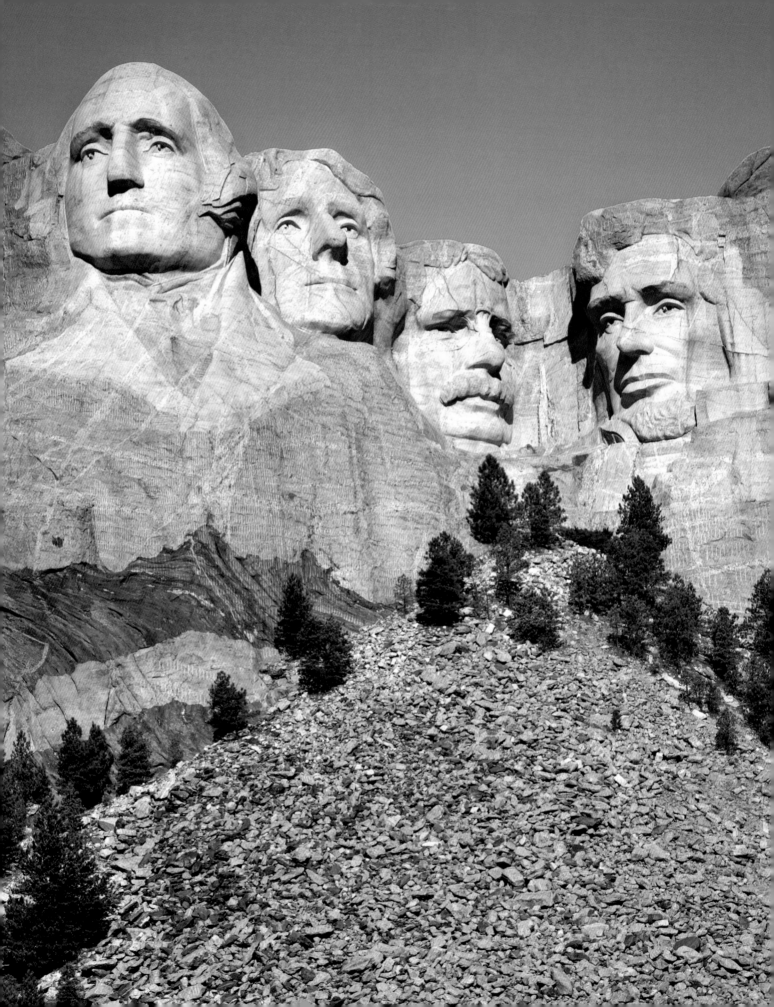

Mount Rushmore

South Dakota

Mount Rushmore's 60-foot busts of Presidents Washington, Jefferson, Roosevelt, and Lincoln were sculpted to represent the first 150 years of American history. They commemorate the birth, growth, preservation, and development of the United States.

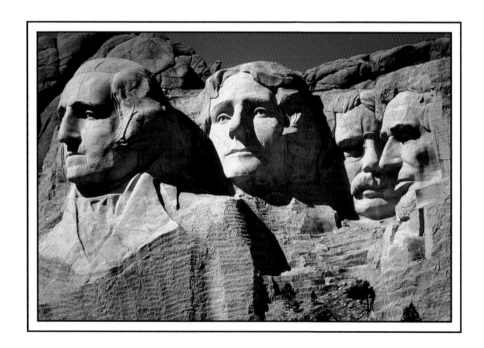

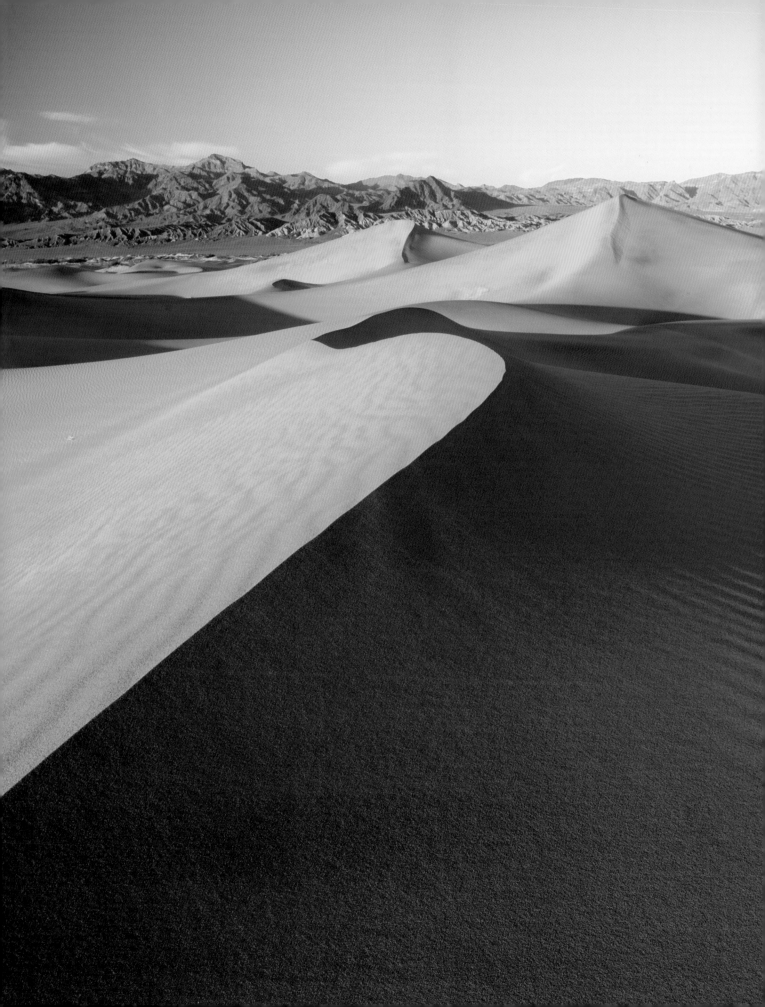

Death Valley

California

Death Valley is located on the border
of California and Nevada. It is the hottest
spot in North America. On July 10th, 1913,
it reached its highest recorded temperature
of 134 degrees Fahrenheit.

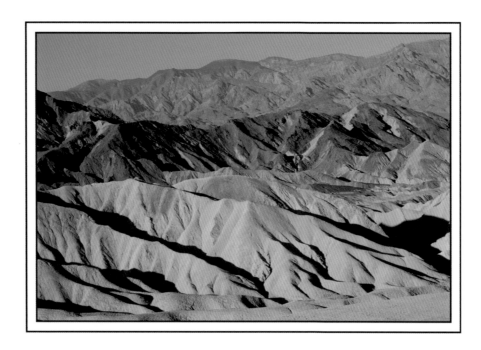

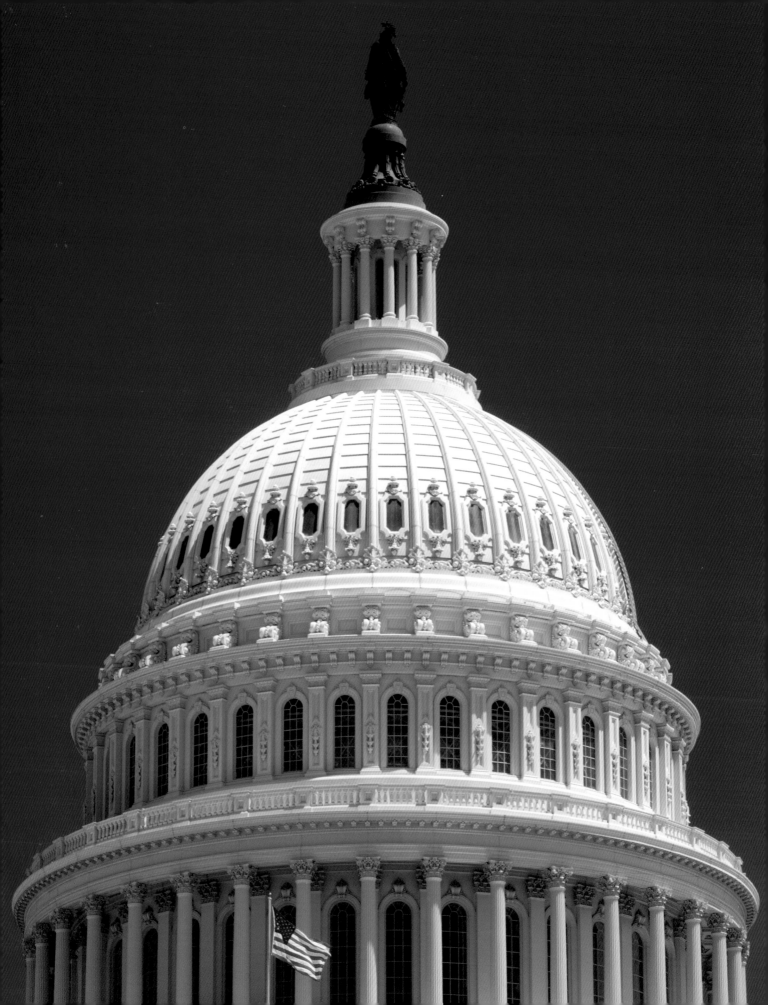

U.S. Capitol Building

Washington, D.C.

The U.S. Capitol Building and its stately dome have become symbols of the American people and democracy. George Washington laid the cornerstone for this, the most important government building in the United States, on September 18th, 1793.

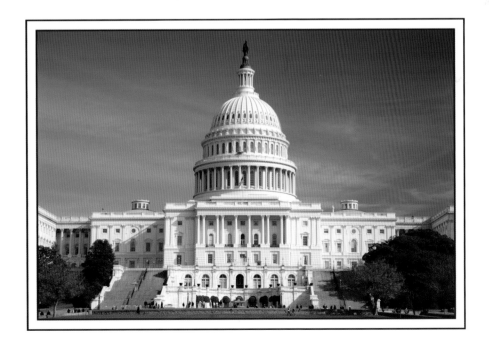

Washington, D.C.

Washington, D.C. is the capital city
of the United States of America.
George Washington chose the site
in preparation for the arrival
of the new government in 1800.
Several government buildings,
monuments, and memorials
are located in Washington, D.C.

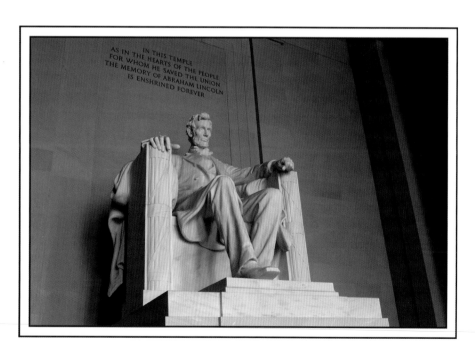

Lincoln Memorial

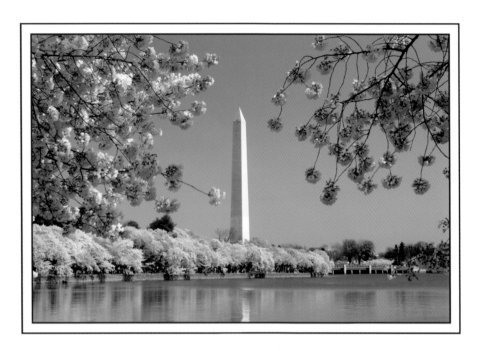

Washington Monument

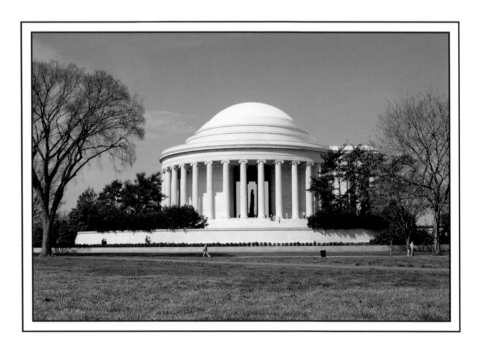

Jefferson Memorial

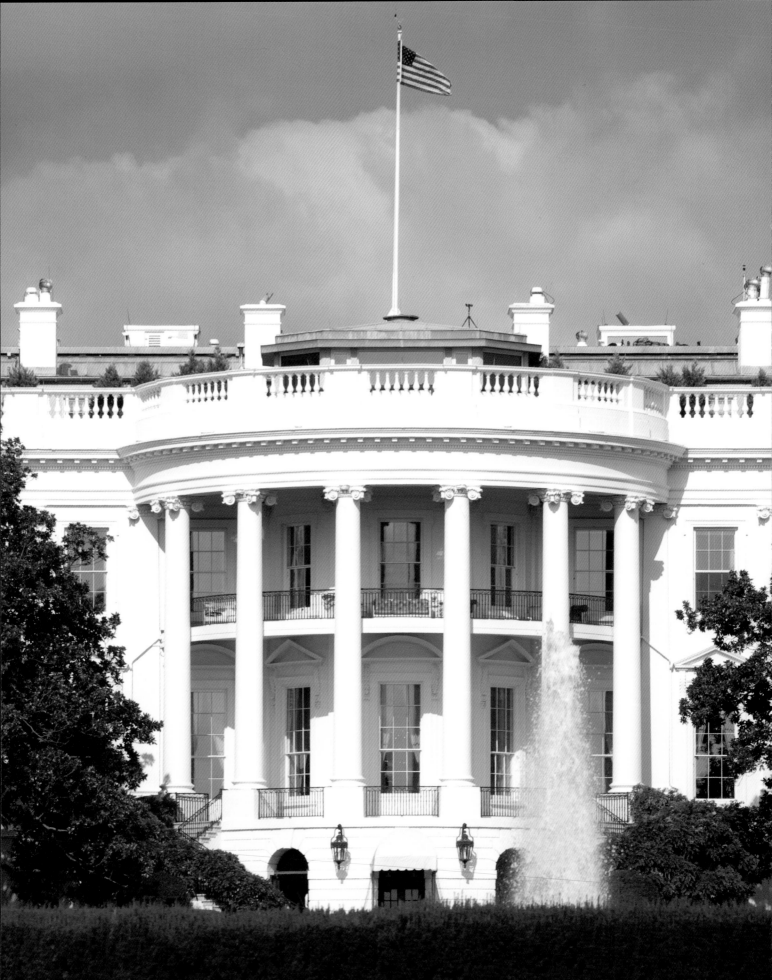

The White House

Washington, D.C.

The White House has stood as a symbol
of the United States Presidency for over
two hundred years. Construction began
in October of 1792, and in 1800
it was occupied by its first residents,
President John Adams and his wife, Abigail.

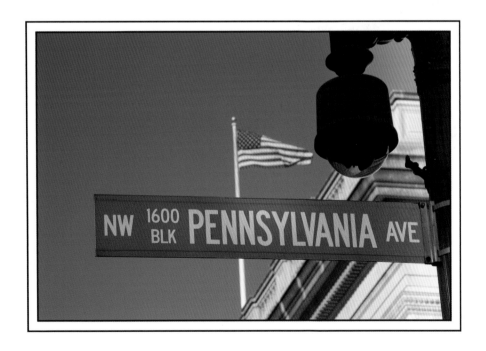

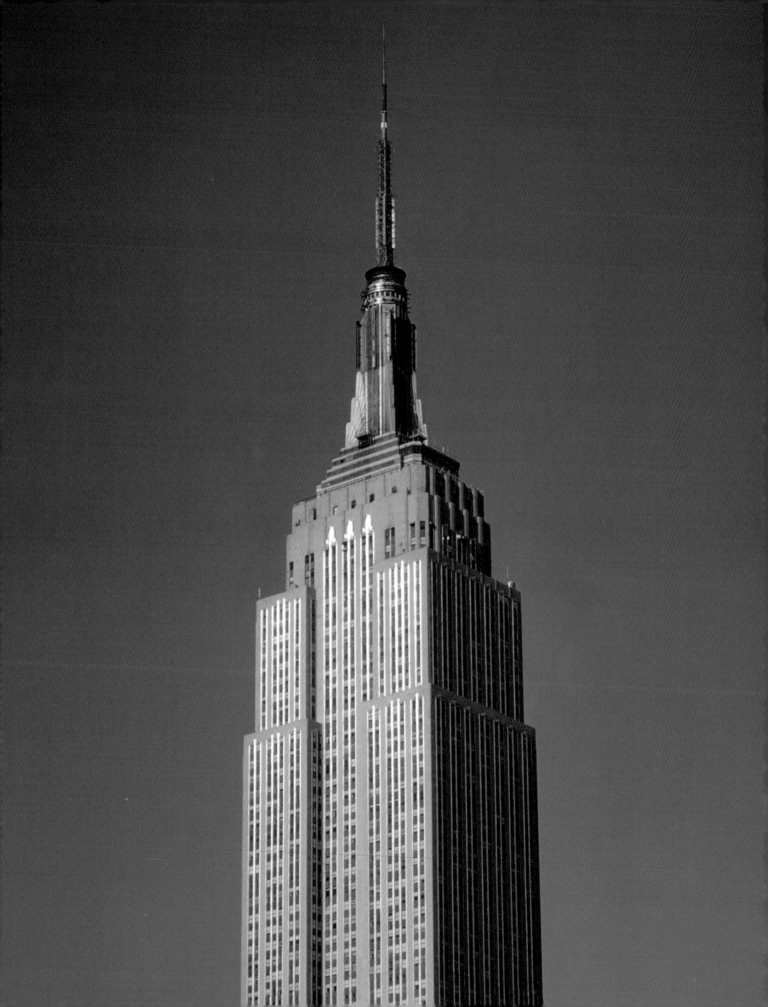

Empire State Building
New York, New York

The Empire State Building is located
at the intersection of Fifth Avenue
and West 34th Street in New York City.
It was completed in 1931, and was
the tallest building in the world
for more than forty years.

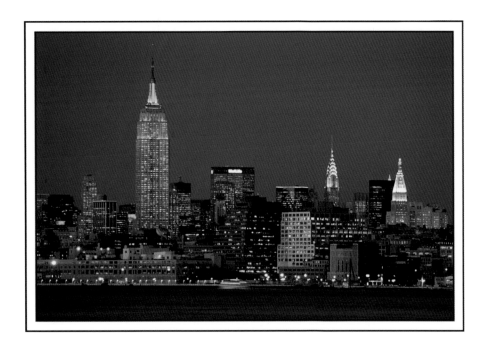

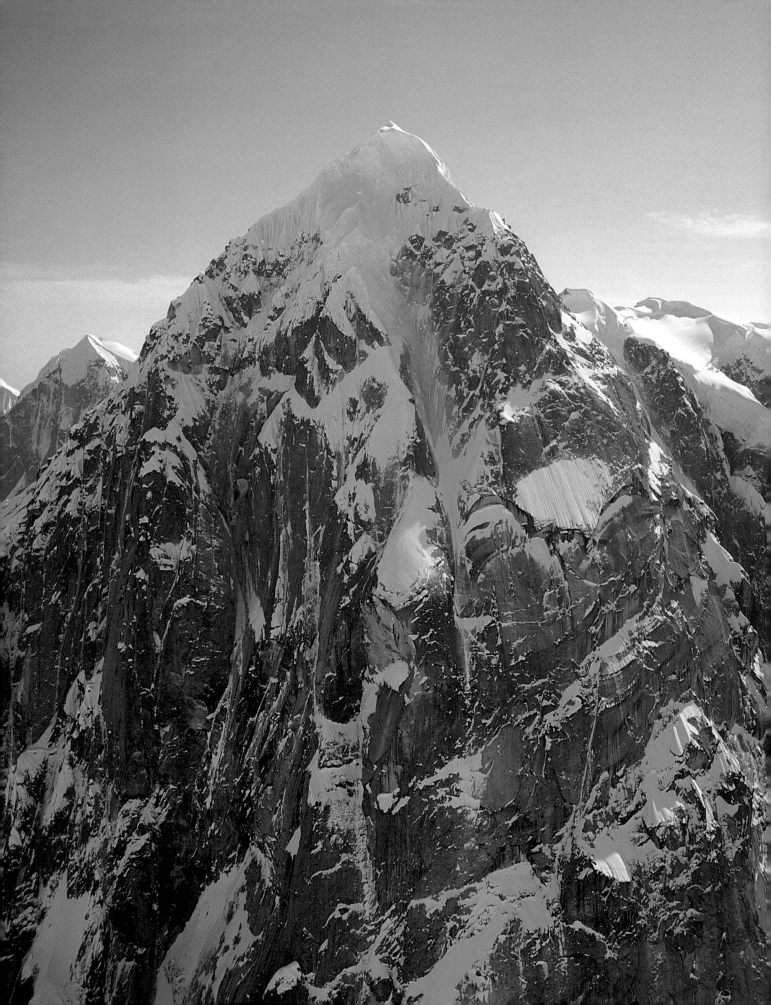

Mount McKinley

Denali National Park, Alaska

Mount McKinley is characterized by its extremely cold weather. With an elevation of 20,320 feet above sea level, it is the highest mountain in North America. Mount McKinley, also known as Denali, was first successfully climbed by a four-man expedition on June 7th, 1913.

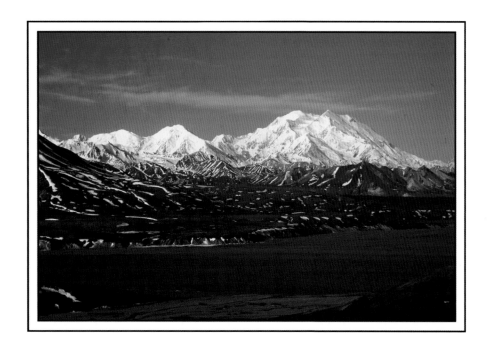

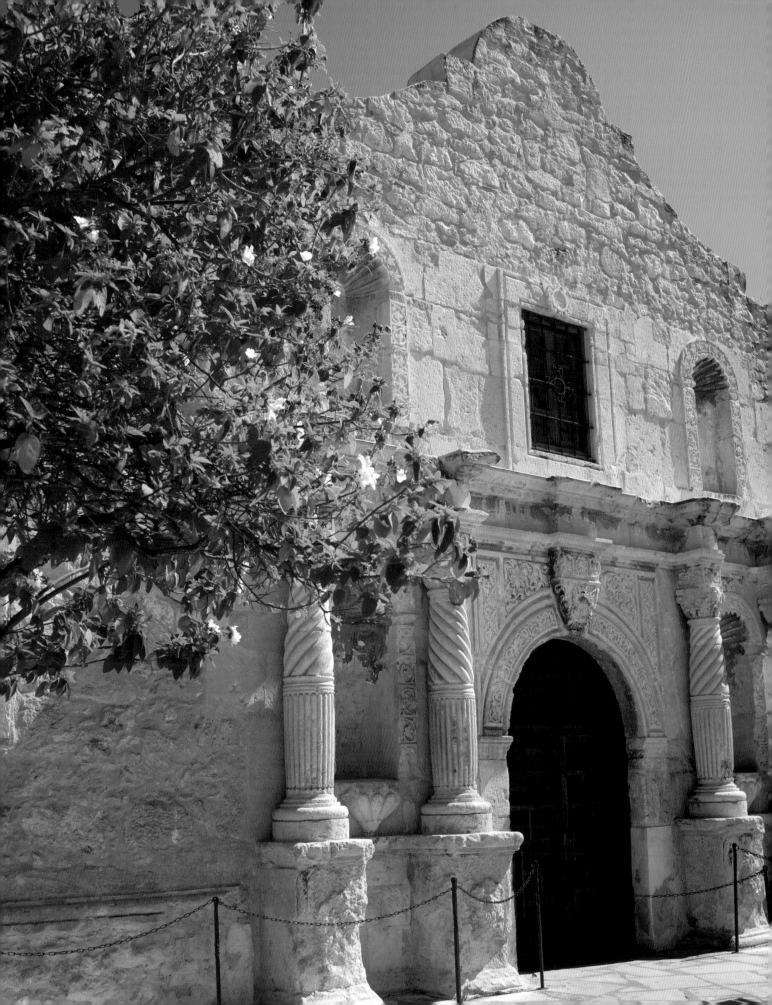

The Alamo

San Antonio, Texas

The Battle of the Alamo was a pivotal point in the Texas Revolution. Although the Texas revolutionaries lost the battle, "Remember the Alamo!" became their battle cry as they successfully won their independence from Mexico on April 21st, 1836.

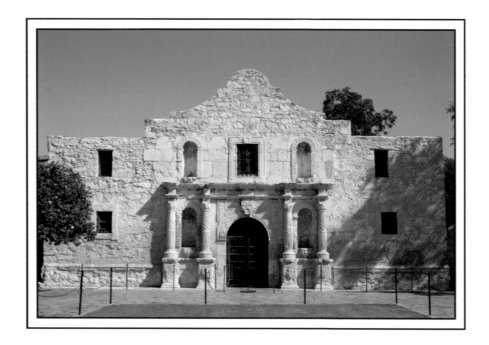

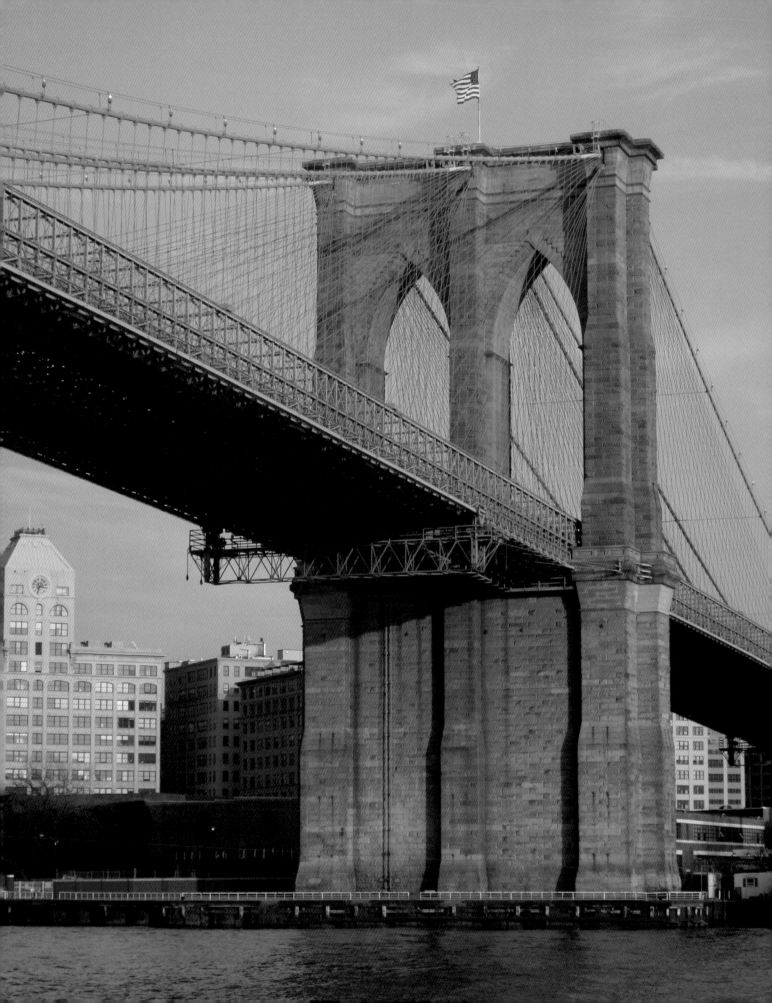

Brooklyn Bridge

New York, New York

The Brooklyn Bridge is one of the oldest suspension bridges in the United States. Completed in 1883, it stretches 5,989 feet over the East River, connecting the boroughs of Manhattan and Brooklyn.

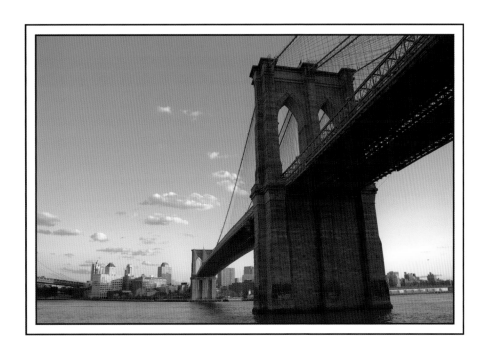

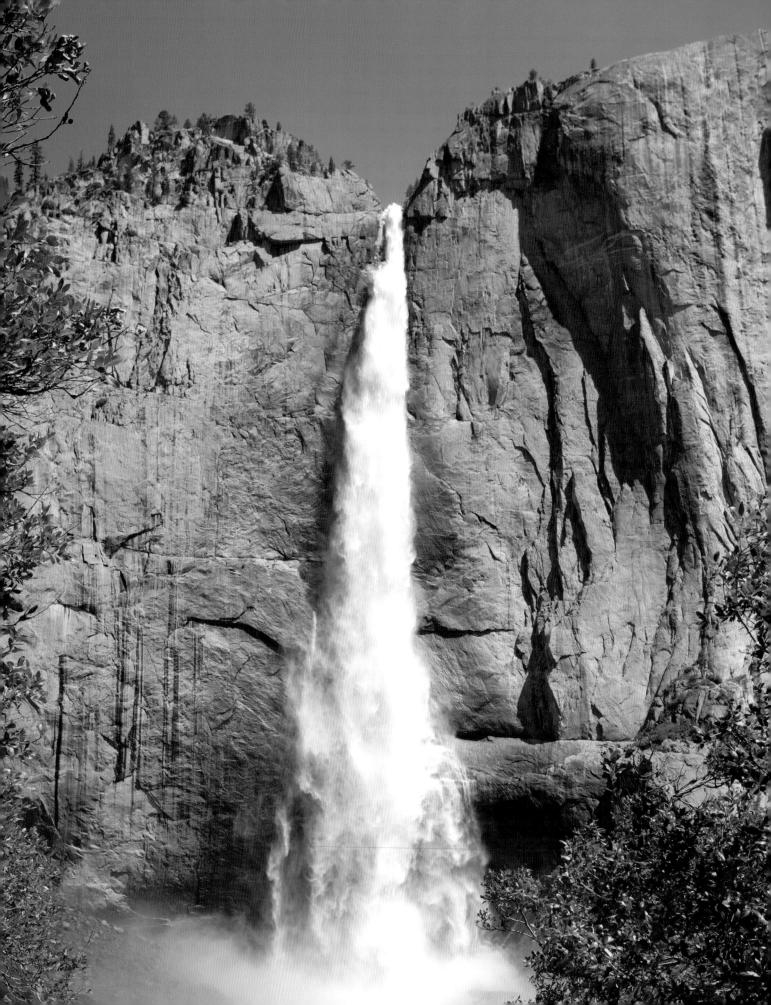

Yosemite National Park
California

Yosemite National Park is best known
for its scenic waterfalls, but its nearly
1,200 square miles is also the home to forests,
meadows, mountain glades, lakes,
and extraordinary views. With 3.5 million
visitors each year, Yosemite is one of America's
most popular parks.

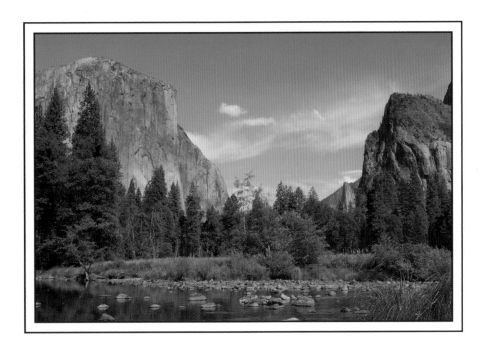

National Parks

America's National Parks are parcels of land owned and managed by the United States government. They are protected from development so that the public can enjoy their wildlife and natural beauty.

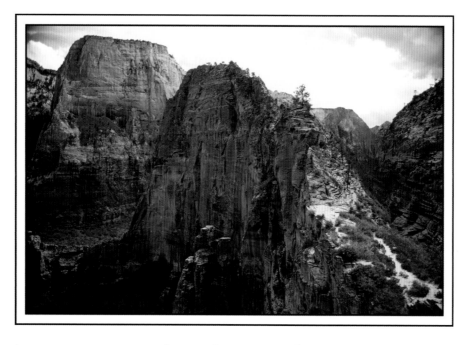

Zion National Park – Utah

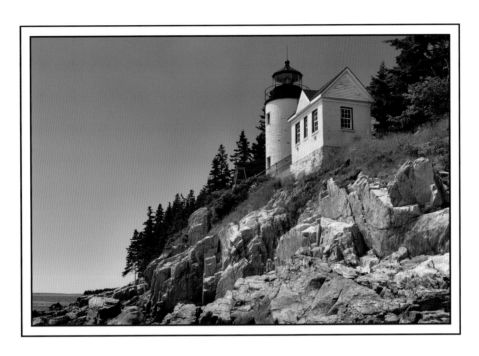

Acadia National Park – Maine

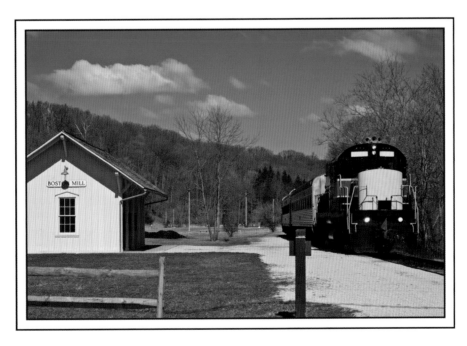

Cuyahoga Valley National Park – Ohio

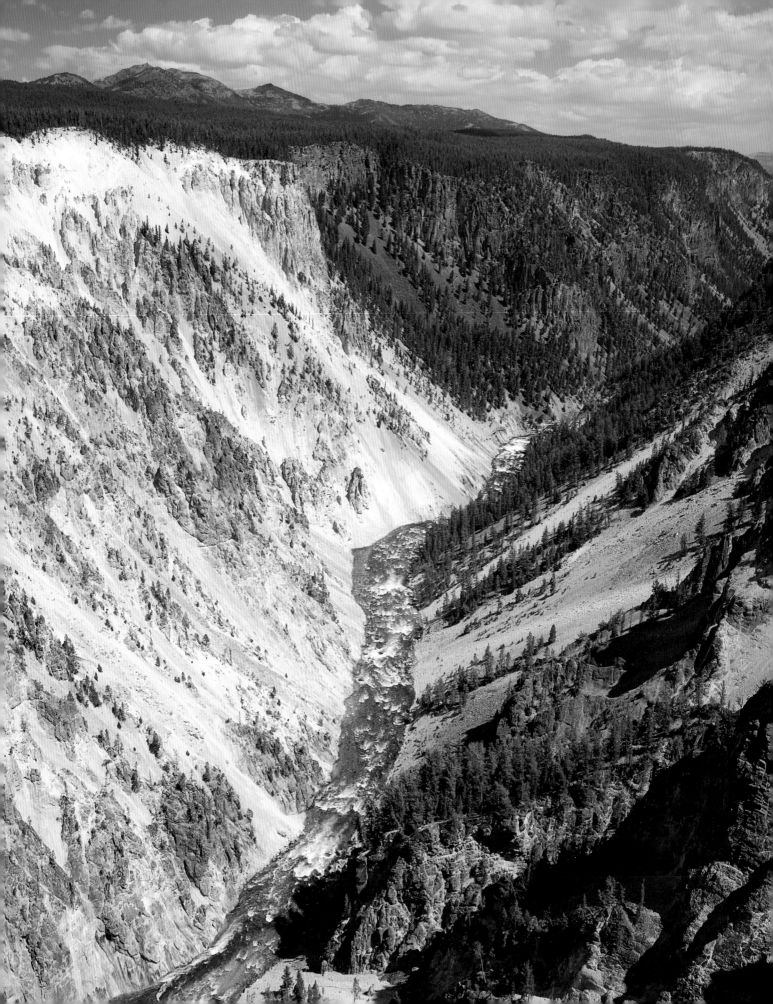

Yellowstone National Park

Wyoming, Montana, Idaho

In 1872, Yellowstone became the first national park established in the United States. It contains nearly 60 percent of the world's geysers, as well as rugged peaks, alpine lakes, deep canyons, and vast forests.

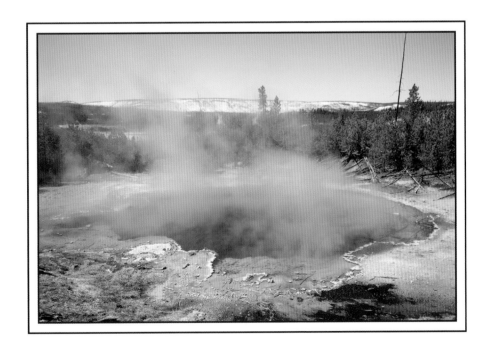

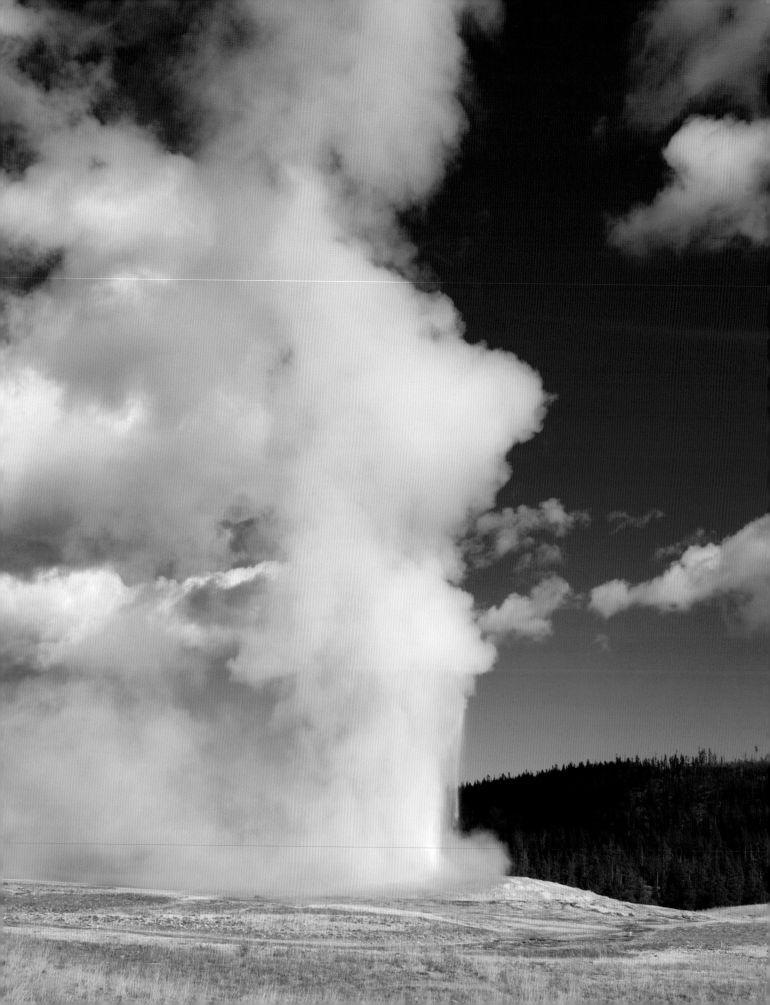

Old Faithful Geyser

Yellowstone National Park, Wyoming

Old Faithful is not the largest or most regular geyser, but it erupts more frequently than any other geyser. It averages 91 minutes between eruptions, which last 1½ to 5 minutes, and reach heights of 90 to 180 feet.

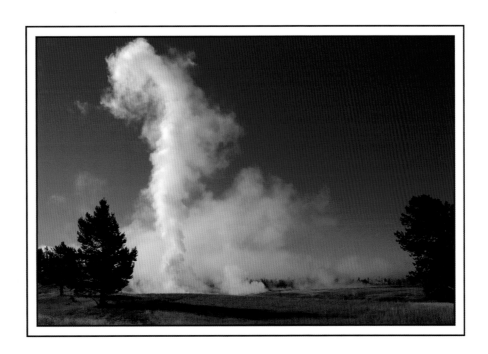

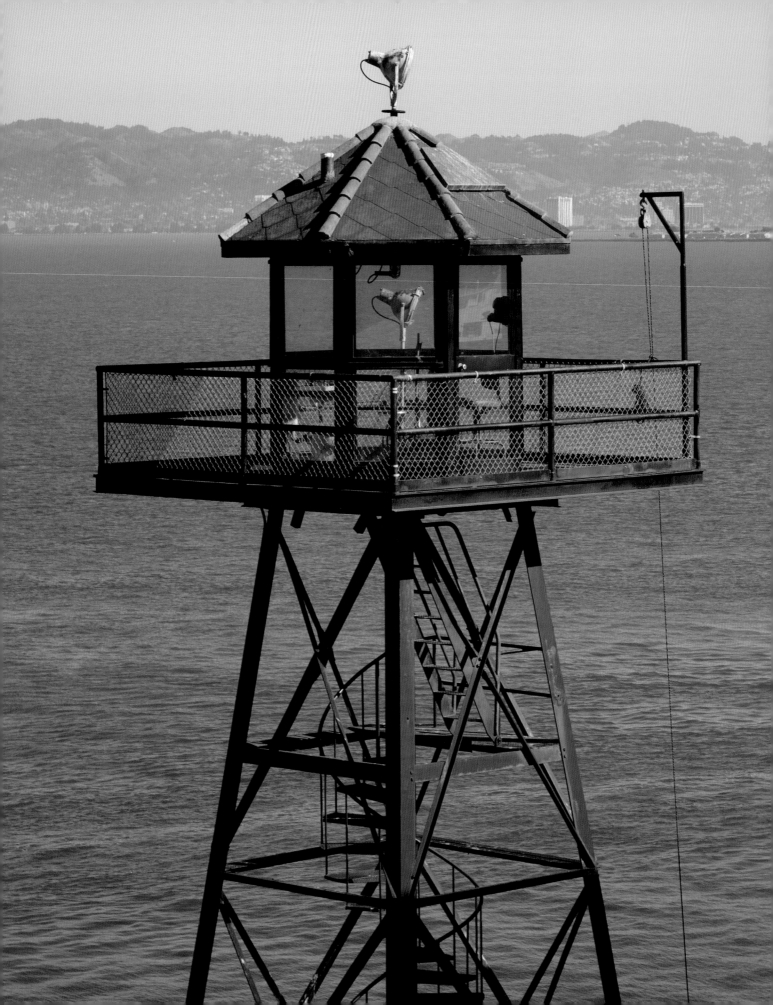

Alcatraz

San Francisco, California

Alcatraz became a federal prison in 1934, housing criminals too dangerous for any other prison. Nicknamed "The Rock," it was an escape-proof prison known for its strict discipline and maximum security.

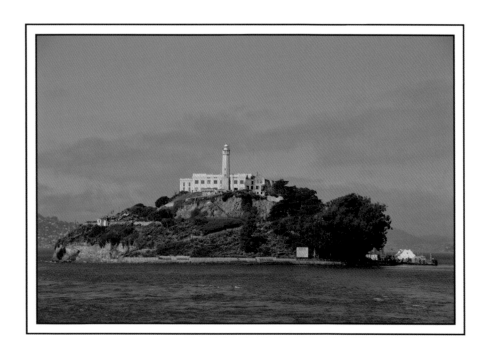

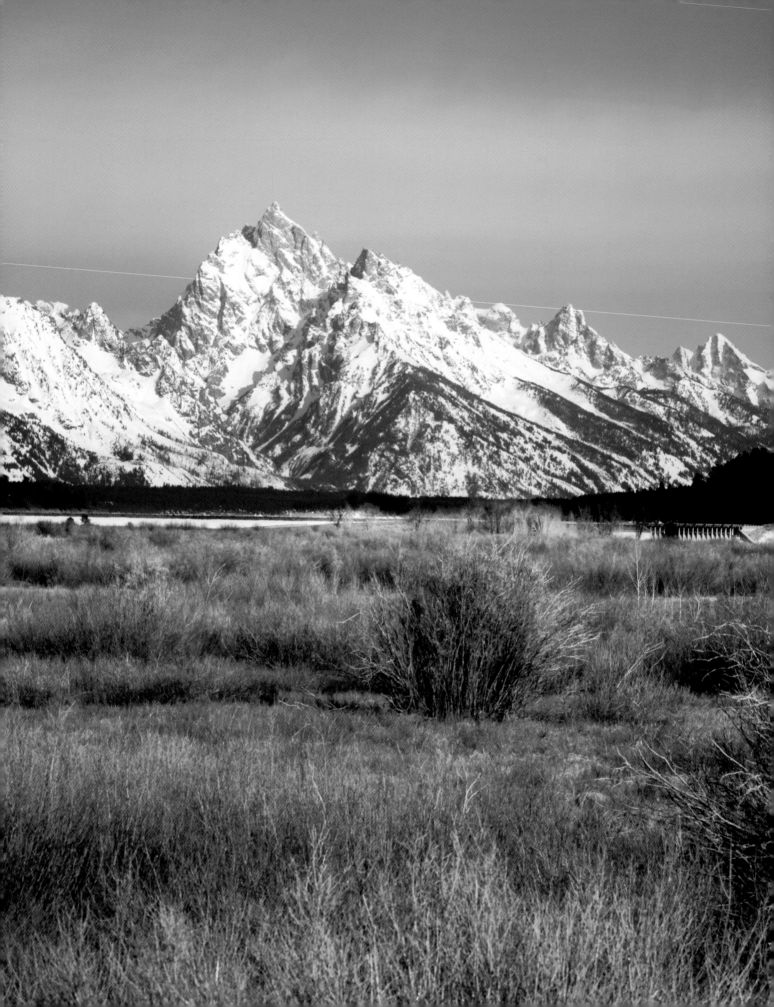

Grand Tetons

Wyoming

The Grand Tetons are located in Wyoming
on the southern side of Yellowstone National Park.
At 13,770 feet above sea level, Grand Teton
is the tallest mountain within the range,
which contains twelve peaks of over 12,000
feet in elevation.

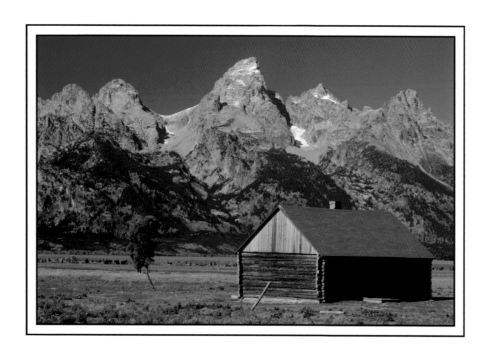

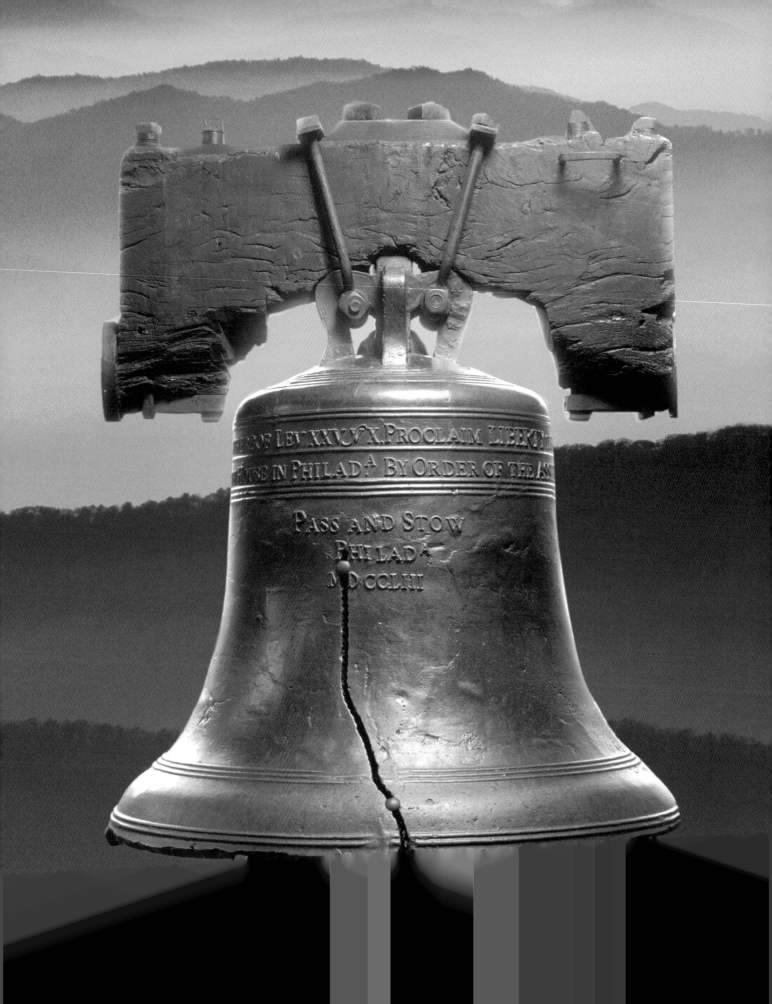

Liberty Bell

Philadelphia, Pennsylvania

The Liberty Bell is a symbol of freedom
in America. On July 8th, 1776, the bell rang
out from the tower of Independence Hall,
summoning citizens to hear the first public
reading of the Declaration of Independence.

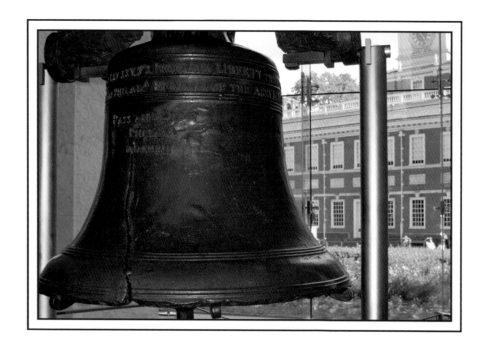

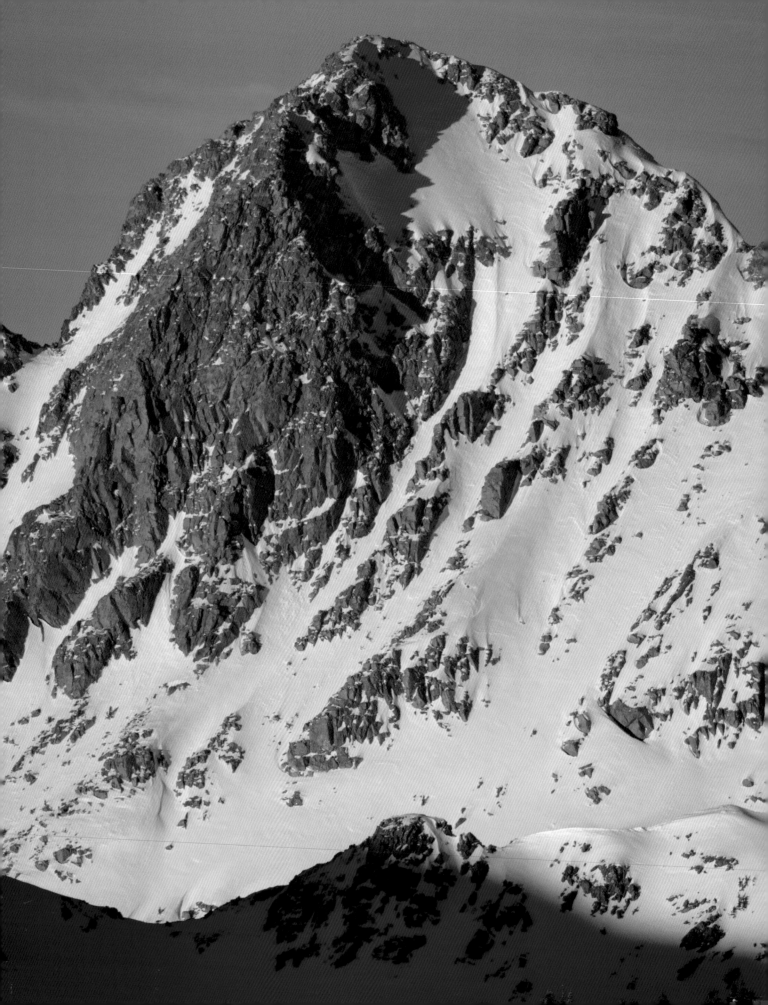

Rocky Mountains

North America

The Rocky Mountains stretch almost 3,000 miles,
from the northernmost part of British Columbia
in Canada, to New Mexico in the United States.
The range's highest peak is Mount Elbert
in central Colorado, at 14,433 feet above sea level.

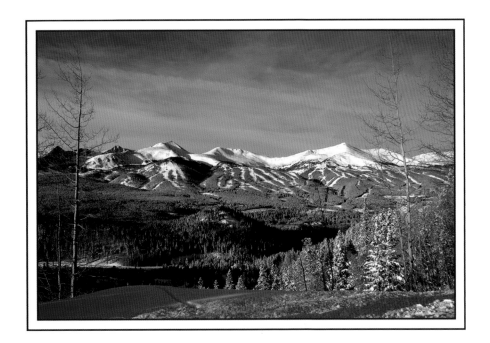

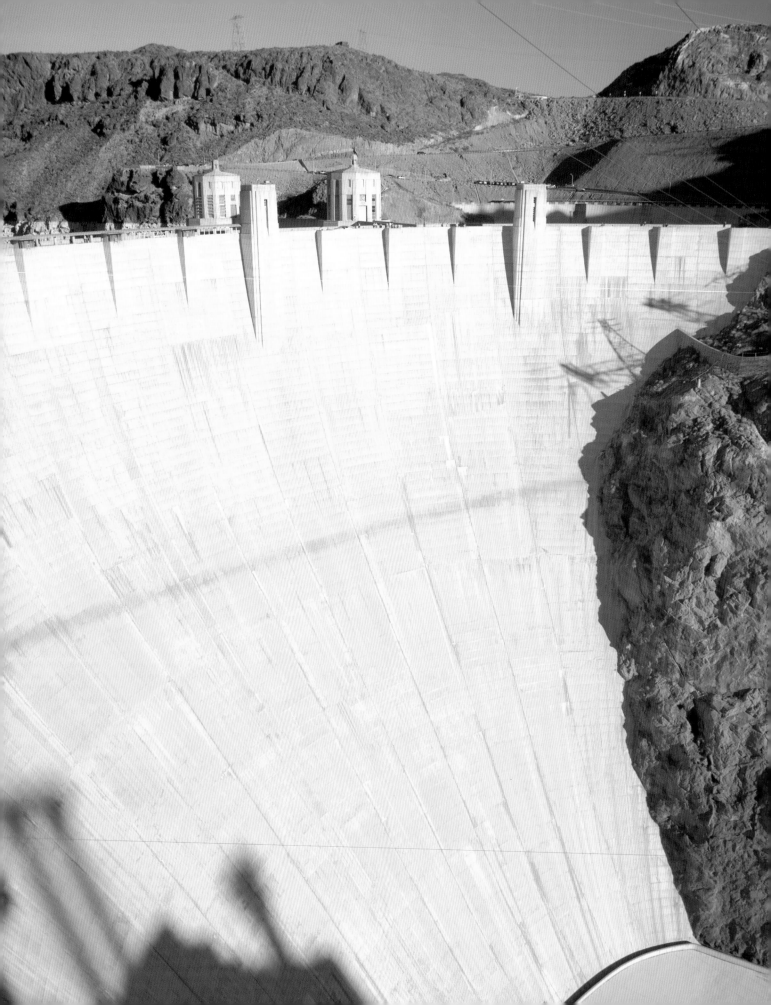

Hoover Dam

Arizona, Nevada

Hoover Dam is located on the Colorado River between Arizona and Nevada. It was completed in 1936, at a cost of 165 million dollars. The dam itself, at 726 feet high, is the tallest concrete dam in the Western Hemisphere.

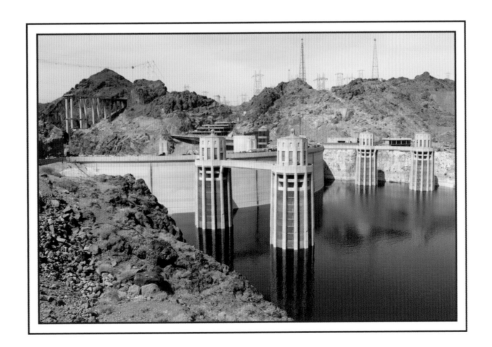

Conversation Starters
and Activities

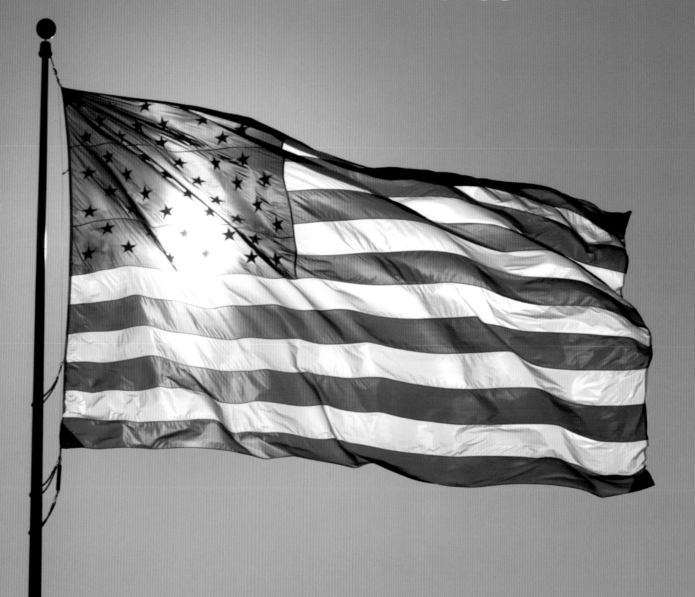

CONVERSATION STARTERS are designed to engage the user and encourage self-expression. They consist of a combination of close-ended (yes or no) and open-ended questions. Each series of four questions correlate to an individual set of pages and are intended to be referenced during the reading experience. Each question is designed to prompt a response by the user from a photograph, word, phrase, or idea from the STORY. After a response from a specific question, either verbal or nonverbal, encourage further discussion on that particular subject. Urging the user to elaborate on an experience allows them to connect to the story and to the caregiver.

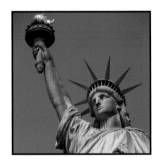

Did you know that the Statue of Liberty is New York City's best known landmark?

Have you ever been to New York City?

Were you born in the United States?

What nationality is your family?

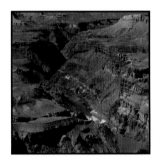

Did you know that at its deepest point, the canyon floor lies over one mile below the rim?

Have you ever gone hiking?

Have you ever traveled by train?

Where did your family go on vacation?

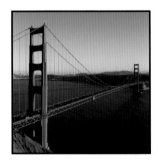

Did you know that the Golden Gate Bridge is the most photographed bridge in the world?

Were there any bridges in your hometown?

Have you ever lived in an area with a lot of fog?

What famous bridges have you driven over?

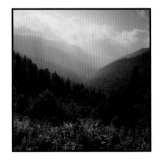

Did you know that the Southern Appalachians are the world's oldest mountain range?

Have you ever stayed overnight in a cabin?

Do you like country music?

Where have you gone hiking?

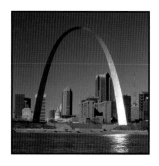

Did you know that the Gateway Arch overlooks the Mississippi River?

Have you ever been on a riverboat?

Do you like blues, jazz, or ragtime music?

What games did you play or songs did you sing on long car trips?

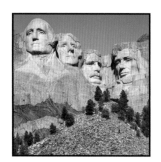

Did you know that multi-colored lights illuminate Niagara Falls at night?

Have you ever been to Niagara Falls?

Have you ever visited Canada?

Who took photographs on your family vacations?

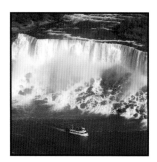

Did you know that Mount Rushmore was sculpted by Gutzon Borglum and over 400 stone workers?

Did you like to study geography when you were in school?

Would you rather stay at a hotel or a campground while on vacation?

Who are some of the U.S. Presidents who served during your lifetime?

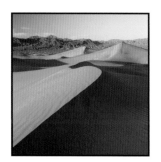

Did you know that spring is the most popular time to visit Death Valley because the wildflowers are in bloom?

Have you ever climbed a sand dune?

Do you prefer to vacation in a warm or cool place?

What kind of flowers bloom in your hometown?

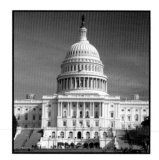

Did you know that the Presidential Inauguration takes place in the Capitol Building?

Have you ever campaigned for a candidate running for office?

Did you like to study U.S. history when you were in school?

What buildings, memorials, or monuments have you visited?

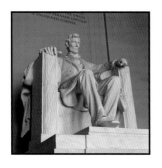

Did you know that the National Cherry Blossom Festival takes place every spring in Washington, D.C.?

Have you ever been to Washington, D.C.?

Did you ever go on a class trip with your schoolmates?

What festivals take place in your hometown?

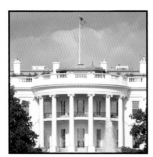

Did you know that the White House and its grounds cover almost 18 acres?

Did you have a yard to play in when you were growing up?

Have you ever seen a rose garden?

Who do you think was the greatest U.S. President?

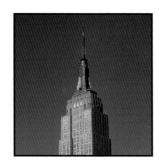

Did you know that the Empire State Building has 102 floors?

Have you ever been in a skyscraper?

Have you ever worked or lived in a tall building?

Where have you traveled by airplane?

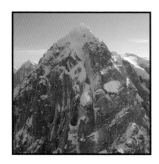

Did you know that Mount McKinley has a recorded low temperature of 75 degrees below zero?

Have you ever been to Alaska?

Do you like the winter months?

What is the furthest distance you have ever traveled?

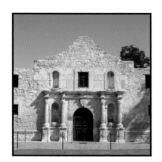

Did you know that the Alamo was originally a Spanish mission run by Franciscan missionaries?

Did your family visit any historical places when you were growing up?

Did you send postcards to family and friends when you vacationed?

What kind of Mexican foods do you like?

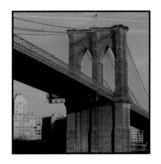

Did you know that before the Brooklyn Bridge was built, the only way to cross the East River was by ferry?

Did you live in a big city or small town when you were growing up?

Have you ever gone shopping in a big city?

What nationalities were common in the neighborhood where you grew up?

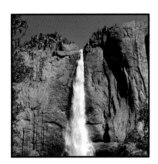

Did you know that Yosemite National Park is home to giant sequoia trees, with some reaching over 300 feet in height?

Have you ever been to Yosemite National Park?

Have you ever put vacation photos in an album?

What time of year did your family go on vacation when you were growing up?

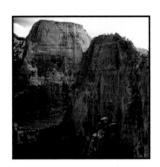

Did you know that the National Parks Service was established in 1916 to manage and regulate the national parks?

Have you ever been to a national park?

Have you ever camped in a national park?

What parks are near your hometown?

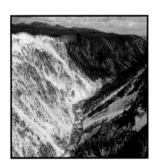

Did you know that Yellowstone National Park has over 200 geysers?

Have you ever gone horseback riding?

Have you ever painted a landscape?

What kind of souvenirs did you buy when you were on vacation?

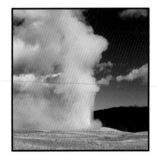

Did you know that Old Faithful has erupted regularly for over 100 years?

Did your family take movies of your vacations?

Have you ever gone on vacation with other families or friends?

What kinds of food do you like to eat on vacation?

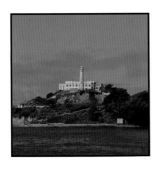

Did you know that officials closed Alcatraz in 1963 because of the high cost of repairs?

Do you like to watch gangster movies?

Have you ever taken a scenic boat ride?

What islands have you visited?

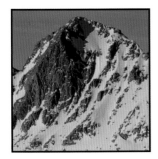

Did you know that the Grand Teton mountain range is 55 miles long?

Have you ever gone snow skiing?

Have you ever gone fishing?

What lakes or streams are near your hometown?

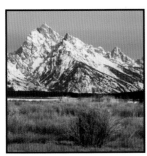

Did you know that the Liberty Bell weighs about 2,000 pounds?

Do you like to watch television shows about travel?

Have you ever attended a family reunion in another state?

How did you and your family celebrate the Fourth of July when you were growing up?

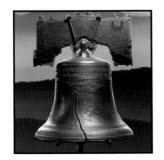

Did you know that Pike's Peak, in the Rocky Mountains, was the inspiration for the song, "America the Beautiful"?

Do you like patriotic songs?

Have you ever driven in the mountains?

What states have you visited?

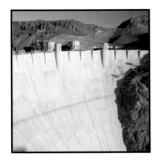

Did you know that Hoover Dam is named after America's 31st President, Herbert Hoover?

Did you like to take guided tours when you were on vacation?

Have you ever lived near a lake or river?

Where did you want to go on vacation when you were a child?

ACTIVITIES are designed to enrich the user's life by introducing diversity into the daily routine through mental and physical engagement. They are intended to be performed under the supervision of a caregiver. Caution should be exercised when outdoors, in unfamiliar surroundings, or when using potentially harmful materials and/or equipment. Selection of an appropriate activity is dependent on individual ability; however, the user may participate or benefit from observing another individual perform the activity.

SENSORY STIMULATION ACTIVITIES

Bake American flag cupcakes. Bake cupcakes and allow them to cool. Top the cupcakes with a white frosting. Add thin pieces of red licorice in a striped pattern and blue sprinkles in the upper-left corner to form the flag design. Enjoy as a dessert on patriotic holidays.

Make a map. Draw a road map of a familiar town. Include the main streets, important landmarks, the school, the library, the grocery store, the firehouse, etc. Label the main streets and prominent locations. Review the map with family and friends.

Sing, hum, or whistle to patriotic songs. Play a variety of well-known patriotic songs and participate in a celebration of America. Experience pride, hope, and love for country, as well as the emotional boost and feelings of well-being that the music provides.

Start a U.S. penny coin collection. Purchase a coin-collecting book for Lincoln cents for the years 1959–2009. Sort through pocket change daily or purchase several rolls of pennies from the bank. Identify the mint dates of coins, place them in the book, and enjoy watching the collection grow.

Keep track of the news. Read a newspaper or watch the televised news daily. Being aware of current events provides topics to discuss when conversing with friends and family.

Build a model car. There are many skill levels of model car kits available, from the simple, no-glue kind to the all-metal, fully customizable types. Purchase a model car kit of an appropriate skill level. Model car building is a fun, relaxing hobby that requires patience and attention to detail.

Visit a rose garden. Roses are one of the oldest known flowers and remain one of the most popular. Locate a local rose garden. Tour several displays of roses, enjoying their majestic beauty and sweet scents while experiencing the grace, elegance, and tranquility of the gardens.

Prepare a regional recipe. Consider preparing a simple dish such as a Philly cheesesteak, shrimp and grits, or Carolina-style barbeque. These dishes are delicious and easy to prepare, and the ingredients are readily available. Enjoy the aroma and authentic flavor of an American favorite.

Study a map of the United States. Look at a map and identify the states resided in and visited. Discuss experiences and adventures, and reminisce about the landscape, the people, and the foods from different locations across the country.

CREATIVE EXPRESSION ACTIVITIES

Make a sand art design. Use a small, clear plastic or glass bottle (or jar) for sand art. Pour a thin layer of colored sand into the container. Add several more layers, alternating different colors of sand. Continue until the container is filled. Place the lid on the container and handle it carefully so the design stays in place.

Create a vacation photo album. Gather a collection of vacation photographs. Arrange the photos on the pages and adhere them using a glue stick. Write a brief description below each photo. Put the finished pages in page protectors and place them in an album. Review the scrapbook and relive memories of good times shared with loved ones.

Paint a landscape. A simple way to paint a landscape is to create rolling hills. Sketch the hills with a few curved lines in pencil on the paper. Paint the sky blue, leaving areas of white to give the illusion of clouds. Paint the hills green, accenting them with yellow or brown. Use a darker shade of green for the hills in the background. Add shrubs along the hills to give the painting a more realistic look.

Create a travel-themed memory box. Decorate a lidded box with vacation photographs, pictures, and embellishments. Fill the box with treasured mementos representing vacations and travel. Guidebooks, tickets, postcards, maps, souvenirs, photographs, etc., may be included. Admire the box and relive special memories of a life story.

PHYSICAL MOVEMENT ACTIVITIES

Plant a "Victory Garden." During World War II, patriotic Americans planted victory gardens consisting of staple vegetables. Determine where to locate the garden. Vegetables need six or more hours of sunlight each day. Plant vegetables that are easy to grow such as lettuce, spinach, carrots, and radishes. Gardening is relaxing, great exercise, and provides the opportunity to get plenty of fresh air and sunshine.

Attend a classic car show. Locate a local classic or antique car show. Watch the owners as they lovingly polish their pride-and-joys. Talk to the owners about their cars. Experience the memories and sense of nostalgia while admiring the vehicles of yesteryear.

Make a rain gauge. Take an empty plastic or glass container and mark ¼ inch graduations from the bottom of the container to the top using a permanent marker. Place the gauge outdoors in an open area. Check the gauge daily and keep a journal to record the amount of rain that is collected each day, week, and month.

Plant a patriotic flower garden. Planting red, white, and blue flowers together is an American tradition. Plant a combination of red, white, and blue petunias or verbenas in the spring. Enjoy the patriotic display on the Fourth of July and all summer long.